I0446200

DASH

DIET COOKBOOK

FOR BEGINNERS 2024

DISCOVER A COLLECTION OF EASY PREP DELICIOUS LOW SODIUM RECIPES FOR A HEART HEALTHY LIFESTYLE.

Marlene E. Martinez

TABLE OF CONTENTS

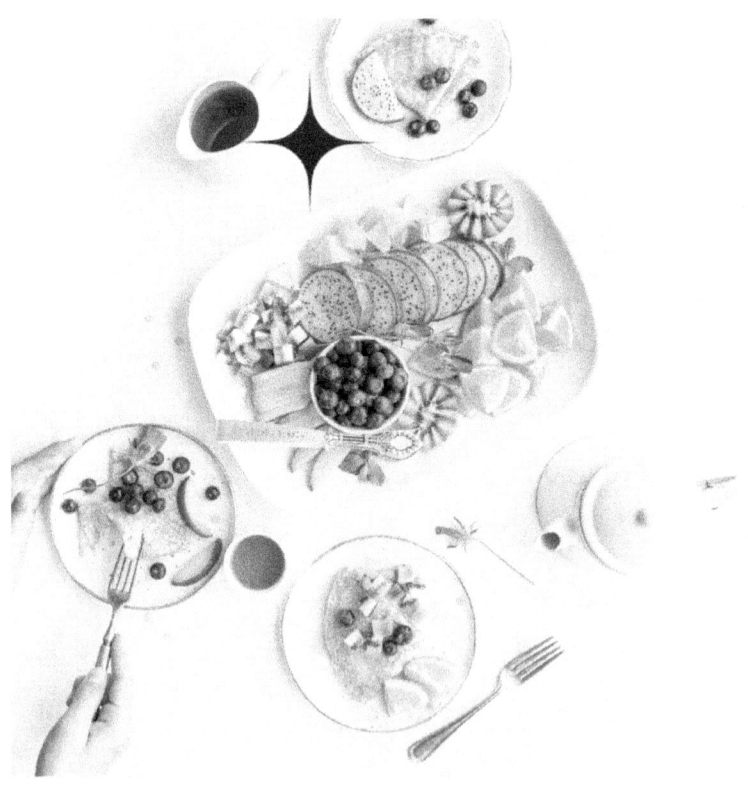

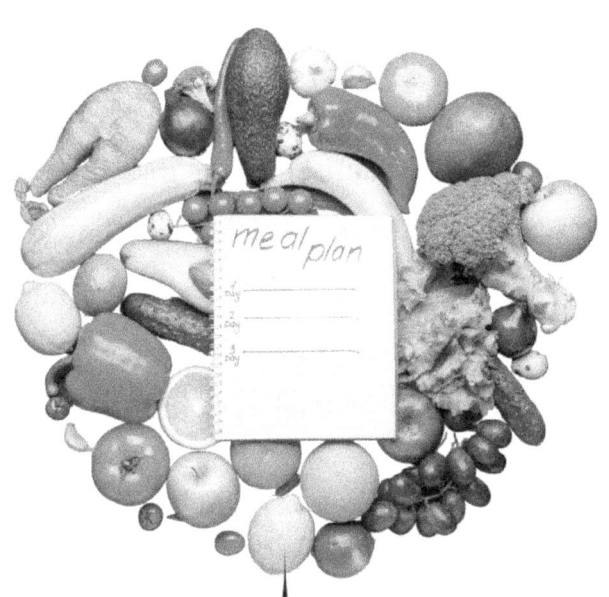

Meal Plan ✔

	Breakfast	Lunch	Dinner
Monday			
Tuesday			
Wednesday			
Thursday			
Friday			
Saturday			
Sunday			

Introduction

Olivia, a devoted chef, lived once upon a time in the busy city of Culinaryville. Olivia was well-known for her cooking skills and ability to turn simple items into spectacular delicacies. While browsing the local bookshop one day, she came across a curious and exciting cookbook titled "Dashing Delights: A Culinary Journey with the Dash Diet."

Olivia was enticed by the promise of delicious and healthful meals and couldn't wait to get her hands on the cookbook. She found the secrets of the DASH (Dietary Approaches to Stop Hypertension) diet as she flipped through the vivid and appealing dishes. The cookbook was a treasure trove of recipes aimed at improving heart health and general well-being.

Olivia chose to start on a culinary adventure after being inspired by the Dash Diet principles. She set out to prepare a meal that would not only satisfy the palate but also nourish the body. Her kitchen was transformed into a laboratory, where she experimented with a wide range of fresh fruits and vegetables, lean proteins, and whole grains.

Olivia's friends and family quickly became willing taste-testers, eagerly awaiting the next delectable item from the Dash Diet cookbook. Her kitchen was filled with the perfume of herbs and spices, and the sizzling noises of sautéing veggies rang throughout her home.

Olivia's wonderful and heart-healthy dinners quickly spread across Culinaryville, catching the attention of a well-known culinary reviewer. The critic paid Olivia a visit because he was intrigued by the idea of a cookbook that combined flavor and nutrition.

As the critic sampled dish after dish, Olivia discussed the Dash Diet's principals and how it had changed her approach to cooking. The culinary critic was astonished not just by the excellent flavors, but also by the dishes' health benefits.

"Dashing Delights" quickly became a Culinaryville sensation, and Olivia's cookbook raced off the shelves. People from many areas of life embraced the Dash Diet, not only as a method of lowering blood pressure, but also as a way of life that recognized the joy of eating well.

As a result, Olivia's experience with the Dash Diet guidebook impacted not only her personal culinary talents, but also the eating patterns of an entire community. The cookbook's pages became a roadmap to a healthier and more flavorful life, demonstrating that the correct ingredients plus a splash of imagination can occasionally create a recipe for success.

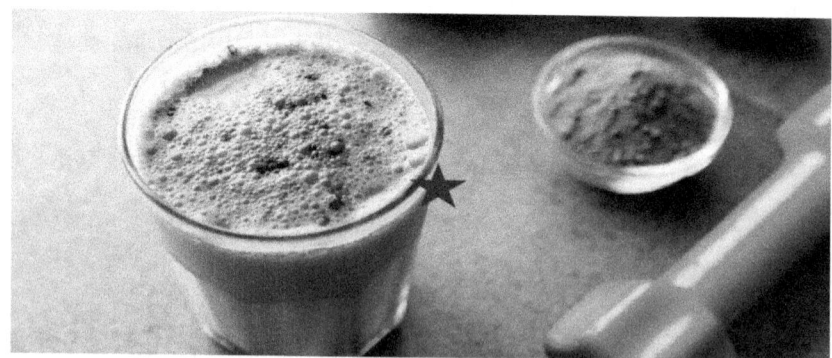

CHAPTER 1: WHAT IS THE DASH DIET?

The DASH diet (Dietary Approaches to Stop Hypertension) is a dietary regimen that is intended to prevent and control hypertension (high blood pressure). The DASH diet, developed by the National Heart, Lung, and Blood Institute (NHLBI), stresses a balanced and heart-healthy approach to eating, with a particular focus on sodium reduction.

DASH Diet Principles:

Focus on Fruits and Vegetables:

The DASH Diet promotes the eating of a wide range of fruits and vegetables that are high in vitamins, minerals, and fiber.

Sources of lean protein:

It encourages the consumption of lean protein sources such as poultry, fish, nuts, and legumes while restricting the consumption of red meat and processed meats.

Grain Whole: Whole grains such as brown rice, quinoa, and whole wheat are preferable than refined grains.

Dairy:

Calcium and vitamin D content in low-fat or fat-free dairy products is emphasized.

Legumes, Nuts, and Seeds:

These were chosen for their nutritional content as well as their supply of healthy fats and protein.

Saturated fat and total fat are limited:

The diet advocates cutting back on saturated and total fats in favor of healthy fats like those found in olive oil or avocados.

Reduced Sodium Consumption:

To assist regulate blood pressure, the DASH Diet recommends decreasing sodium intake. This includes lowering the amount of salt used in cooking and avoiding high-sodium manufactured foods.

Benefits of the DASH Diet

The DASH diet (Dietary Approaches to Stop Hypertension) is a well-researched dietary regimen aimed at preventing and managing hypertension (high blood pressure). The following are some of the advantages of the DASH diet:

Blood Pressure Control: The DASH diet's major purpose is to effectively lower and manage blood pressure, making it a good choice for people who have hypertension.

Cardiovascular Health: Reduces the risk of heart disease and stroke, promoting cardiovascular health.

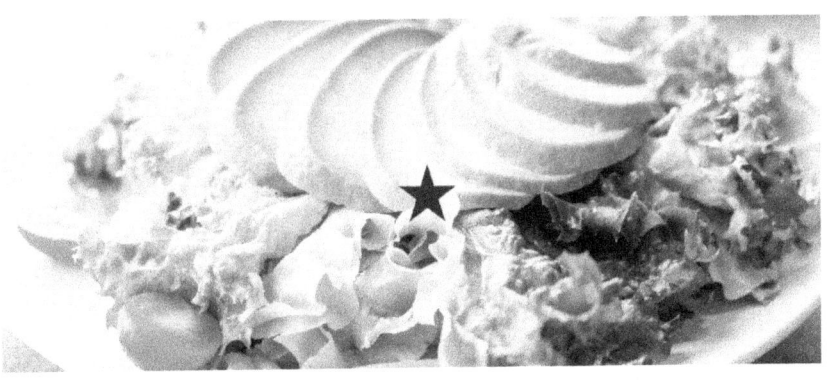

Nutrition that is well-balanced: Encourages the eating of a range of foods from various food groups to promote a balanced and nutrient-rich diet.

Potassium-rich foods include: The DASH diet is strong in potassium, which can help balance sodium's effects on blood pressure and contribute to overall heart health.

Reduced Sodium Consumption: Reduces sodium consumption, which is important for controlling blood pressure and lowering the risk of cardiovascular events.

Weight Control: Supports weight loss and management by emphasizing full, nutrient-dense diets and portion control.

Lower Cholesterol Levels: Can aid in the reduction of LDL (bad) cholesterol levels and the improvement of overall cholesterol profiles.

Diabetes Control: Diabetes patients may benefit from improved blood sugar control and insulin sensitivity.

Fiber-rich foods: The diet is high in fiber, which promotes digestive health, aids in weight maintenance, and may lower the chance of acquiring certain chronic illnesses.

Chronic Disease Risk is Reduced: The DASH diet has been linked to a lower risk of chronic diseases such type 2 diabetes, some malignancies, and osteoporosis.

Increased Consumption of Nutrient-Rich Foods: Encourages the consumption of fruits, vegetables, lean proteins, whole grains, and low-fat dairy, all of which provide important nutrients for overall health.

Flexibility: The DASH diet is versatile and may be customized to match individual preferences and nutritional demands, making it long-term adherence possible.

Encourages Healthy Eating Habits: Encourages conscious eating and the establishment of long-lasting good eating habits.

Promotes Overall Well-Being: The combination of balanced nutrition and lifestyle advice adds to general well-being improvement.

Scientifically Supported: Extensive scientific evidence backs up the DASH diet, which has been recommended by health organizations as an effective dietary approach for blood pressure management.

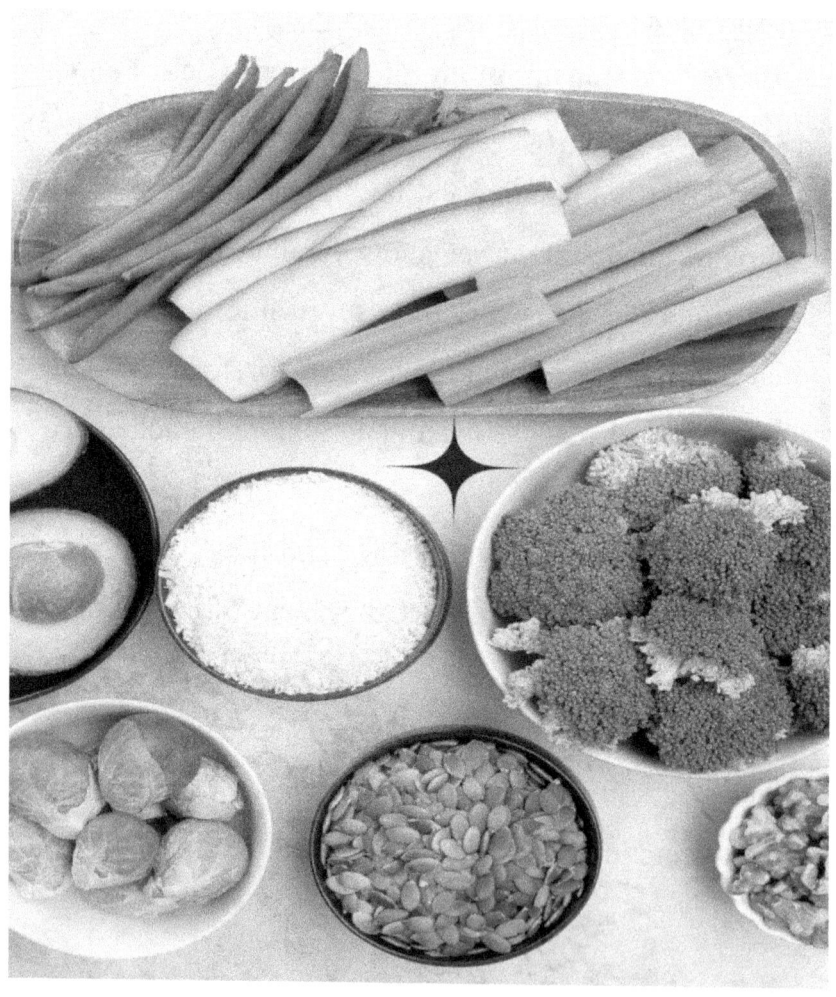

CHAPTER 2: BREAKFAST DELIGHTS

Greek Yogurt Parfait:

Ingredients:

- 2 cups plain non-fat Greek yogurt
- 1 cup fresh mixed berries (strawberries, blueberries, raspberries)
- 1/2 cup granola (low-sugar, whole grain)
- 1/4 cup chopped nuts (almonds, walnuts)
- 1 tablespoon honey or maple syrup (optional)
- 1 teaspoon vanilla extract
- 1/2 teaspoon cinnamon

Prep Time: 10 minutes

Quantity: Makes 2 servings

Preparation:

1. In a mixing dish, combine the Greek yogurt, vanilla extract, and cinnamon.

2. Layer the Greek yogurt mixture with fresh mixed berries in serving cups or bowls.
3. Sprinkle granola and chopped nuts over the layers of yogurt and berries.
4. If desired, drizzle with honey or maple syrup to add sweetness.
5. Repeat the layers until the glass or bowl is full, finishing with a granola and nut sprinkle on top.
6. Enjoy your tasty and healthful Greek Yogurt Parfait right away!

Oatmeal with Fruit:

Ingredients:

- 1 cup old-fashioned oats
- 2 cups water
- 1/2 teaspoon cinnamon
- 1/4 teaspoon salt
- 1 cup mixed berries (strawberries, blueberries, raspberries)
- 1 medium banana, sliced
- 2 tablespoons chopped nuts (walnuts, almonds)

- 1 tablespoon chia seeds
- 1 cup skim milk or unsweetened almond milk
- 1 teaspoon honey or maple syrup (optional for sweetness)

Preparation Time:15 minutes

Quantity:2 servings

Instructions:

1. Cooking Oats:

Bring 2 cups of water to a boil in a medium-sized pot.

Reduce the heat to low and stir in 1 cup of old-fashioned oats.

Stir in the cinnamon and salt and cook for about 10 minutes, or until the oats are soft.

2. Prepare the fruits:

Wash and slice the berries and banana while the oats are cooking.

3. Assemble:

Divide the cooked oats evenly between two bowls.

Add a dollop of mixed berries, banana slices, and chopped nuts to each bowl.

4. Optional Extras:

Each bowl should have 1 tablespoon of chia seeds.

5. Pour the milk:

Over each bowl, pour 1/2 cup skim milk or unsweetened almond milk.

6. (Optional): sweeten

To add sweetness, sprinkle 1/2 teaspoon honey or maple syrup over each bowl.

7. Serve:

Combine the ingredients and serve the oatmeal warm.

Whole Grain Toast with Avocado:

Ingredients:

- 2 slices of whole grain bread
- 1 ripe avocado
- 1 tablespoon lemon juice
- Salt and pepper to taste
- Optional toppings: cherry tomatoes, red pepper flakes, or a sprinkle of chia seeds

Prep Time: 10 minutes

Quantity: 2 servings

Instructions:

1. Toast the whole grain bread as follows:

Toast the whole grain bread slices to your preferred level of doneness.

2. To make the avocado spread, follow these steps:

Cut the avocado in half, remove the pit, and spoon the flesh into a bowl as the bread toasts.

Mash the avocado with a fork until it reaches the desired smoothness.

To taste, add lemon juice, salt, and pepper. Combine thoroughly.

3. Prepare the Toast:

After toasting the bread, distribute the mashed avocado equally over each piece.

4. Optional Extras:

To add taste and nutrients, garnish with sliced cherry tomatoes, a sprinkling of red pepper flakes, or a sprinkle of chia seeds.

5. Serve:

While the bread is still warm, serve the Whole Grain Toast with Avocado right away.

Vegetable Omelette:

Ingredients:

- 2 large eggs
- 1/4 cup diced bell peppers (assorted colors)
- 1/4 cup diced tomatoes
- 2 tablespoons diced red onion
- 1/4 cup chopped spinach
- 1/4 cup diced zucchini
- 1/4 teaspoon black pepper
- 1/4 teaspoon garlic powder
- 1/4 teaspoon onion powder
- 1/4 teaspoon dried oregano
- 1/4 teaspoon dried basil
- 1/4 teaspoon salt (optional)
- 1 teaspoon olive oil

Preparation Time:10 minutes

Quantity:1 serving

Instructions:

1. In a mixing basin, thoroughly combine the eggs.

2. In a nonstick skillet over medium heat, heat the olive oil.

3. To the skillet, add diced bell peppers, tomatoes, red onion, spinach, and zucchini. Sauté for 3-5 minutes, or until vegetables are soft.

4. Season the sautéed vegetables with black pepper, garlic powder, onion powder, dried oregano, and dried basil. To blend, stir everything together.

5. Pour the beaten eggs over the vegetables in the skillet, making sure they're evenly distributed.

6. Allow the eggs to set around the edges before serving. Lift the edges gently with a spatula to allow raw eggs to run to the edges.

7. Fold the omelette in half with a spatula once it is mostly set but still somewhat runny on top.

8. Cook for a another 1-2 minutes, or until the eggs are thoroughly cooked and the vegetables are soft.

9. Transfer the omelette to a platter and season with salt to taste.

10. Enjoy your tasty and nutritious DASH diet-friendly Vegetable Omelette while it's still hot!

Quinoa Breakfast Bowl:

Ingredients:

- 1 cup quinoa, rinsed
- 2 cups water
- 1 cup skim milk or unsweetened almond milk
- 1 teaspoon vanilla extract
- 1 tablespoon honey or maple syrup (optional)
- 1 cup mixed berries (strawberries, blueberries, raspberries)
- 1 medium banana, sliced
- 1 tablespoon chia seeds
- 1 tablespoon chopped nuts (walnuts, almonds, or your choice)
- 1/2 teaspoon cinnamon
- Greek yogurt for topping (optional)

Preparation Time:15 minutes

Quantity:2 servings

Instructions:

1. Quinoa Cooking Instructions:

Combine quinoa and water in a medium saucepan. Bring to a boil, then reduce to a low heat, cover, and cook for 12-15 minutes, or until the quinoa is tender and the water has been absorbed.

2. Make the Quinoa Base:

When the quinoa is done, fluff it with a fork.

Warm the milk in a separate pot over medium heat. If using, add the vanilla essence and honey or maple syrup. Stir until thoroughly blended.

Stir together the milk mixture and the cooked quinoa.

3. Make the Breakfast Bowl:

Divide the quinoa mixture evenly between two dishes.

Top each bowl with a mixture of berries, banana slices, chia seeds, chopped almonds, and cinnamon.

4. Optional Extras:

If preferred, top with a dollop of Greek yogurt.

5. Serve:

Serve the Quinoa Breakfast Bowl right away for a healthful and filling breakfast.

Smoothie Bowl:

Ingredients:

- 1 cup fresh berries (strawberries, blueberries, raspberries)
- 1 medium banana, sliced
- 1/2 cup Greek yogurt (low-fat or fat-free)
- 1/4 cup old-fashioned oats
- 1 tablespoon chia seeds
- 1/2 cup skim milk or almond milk
- 1 teaspoon honey (optional for sweetness)
- 1/4 cup nuts (almonds, walnuts) for topping
- 1 tablespoon flaxseeds for topping
- Fresh mint leaves for garnish (optional)

Prep Time:15 minutes

Quantity:1 serving

Instructions:

1. Blend together the fresh berries, sliced banana, Greek yogurt, old-fashioned oats, chia seeds, and milk in a blender.

2. Blend until the mixture is smooth and creamy. If the mixture is too thick, add more milk to achieve the appropriate consistency.

3. If you prefer a sweeter flavor, add honey to the smoothie. Blend one more to incorporate the honey.

4. Fill a bowl halfway with the smoothie.

5. To add texture and taste, top the smoothie bowl with almonds, flaxseeds, and fresh mint leaves.

6. Enjoy your tasty and healthy Dash Diet Smoothie Bowl!

Whole Wheat Pancakes:

Ingredients:

- 1 cup whole wheat flour
- 1 tablespoon sugar
- 1 teaspoon baking powder
- 1/2 teaspoon baking soda
- 1/4 teaspoon salt
- 1 cup low-fat milk
- 1 large egg

- 2 tablespoons vegetable oil
- Cooking spray or additional oil for greasing the pan

Preparation Time:15 minutes

Quantity: Makes about 8-10 pancakes

Instructions:

1. Whisk together the whole wheat flour, sugar, baking powder, baking soda, and salt in a large mixing basin.

2. In a separate bowl, whisk together the egg, milk, and vegetable oil. Combine thoroughly.

3. Stir the wet components into the dry ingredients until they are barely mixed. Make sure not to overmix; a few lumps are fine.

4. Over medium-high heat, heat a griddle or nonstick skillet. Cooking spray or a tiny amount of oil should be lightly coated.

5. For each pancake, pour 1/4 cup batter onto a hot griddle. Cook until surface bubbles appear, then

flip and cook until the second side is golden brown.

6. Repeat until all of the batter has been utilized.

Chia Seed Pudding:

Ingredients:

- 1/4 cup chia seeds
- 1 cup unsweetened almond milk (or any milk of your choice)
- 1/2 teaspoon vanilla extract
- 1 tablespoon honey or maple syrup (optional, depending on your sweetness preference)
- 1/2 cup mixed berries (strawberries, blueberries, raspberries) for topping
- 1 tablespoon chopped nuts (almonds, walnuts) for topping

Preparation Time:5 minutes (plus additional time for chilling)

Quantity:2 servings

Instructions

1. In a mixing dish, combine the chia seeds, almond milk, vanilla extract, and honey or maple syrup (if using). To blend, stir everything together thoroughly.

2. Allow the mixture to sit for a few minutes before stirring again to prevent clumping.

3. Refrigerate the bowl for at least 2 hours or overnight to allow the chia seeds to absorb the liquid and form a pudding-like consistency.

4. Stir the pudding well before serving to break up any clumps and achieve a smooth texture.

5. Divide the chia seed pudding into two glasses or bowls.

6. Add a handful of mixed berries and a sprinkling of chopped nuts to each serving.

7. Enjoy your nutritious Dash Diet Chia Seed Pudding cold!

Breakfast Burrito:

Ingredients:

- 2 whole wheat tortillas (6-inch)
- 4 large eggs, beaten
- 1 cup diced tomatoes
- 1/2 cup black beans, drained and rinsed
- 1/2 cup diced bell peppers (any color)
- 1/4 cup diced red onion
- 1/4 cup shredded low-fat cheddar cheese
- 1 tablespoon olive oil
- 1 teaspoon ground cumin
- 1/2 teaspoon garlic powder
- Salt and pepper to taste
- Fresh cilantro for garnish (optional)
- Salsa or hot sauce for serving (optional)

Prep Time:15 minutes

Quantity:2 servings

Instructions:

1. In a skillet over medium heat, heat the olive oil.

2. To the skillet, add diced red onion and bell peppers. 3-4 minutes, or until vegetables are soft.

3. To the skillet, add black beans and diced tomatoes. Cook for another 2 minutes, stirring occasionally.

4. Pour the beaten eggs into one side of the skillet and the veggie mixture into the other.

5. Season the eggs with cumin, garlic powder, salt, and pepper to taste. Scramble the eggs until they are completely done.

6. When the eggs have finished cooking, combine them with the veggie mixture in the skillet.

7. Warm the whole wheat tortillas for about 15 seconds in a dry skillet or in the microwave.

8. Divide the egg and veggie mixture among the two tortillas evenly.

9. Sprinkle shredded cheese on top of each tortilla's filling.

10. To make a burrito, roll up the tortillas and fold in the sides.

11. If desired, garnish with fresh cilantro.

12. If desired, serve with salsa or hot sauce on the side.

Fruit Salad with Cottage Cheese:

Ingredients:

- 2 cups fresh strawberries, hulled and sliced
- 1 cup fresh blueberries
- 1 cup fresh pineapple, diced
- 1 cup fresh mango, diced
- 1 cup seedless grapes, halved
- 1 cup low-fat cottage cheese
- 2 tablespoons honey (optional, for drizzling)
- Fresh mint leaves for garnish (optional)

Preparation Time:15 minutes

Quantity:4 servings

Instruction:

Wash and prep all of the fresh fruits listed in the ingredient list.

1. Fruits to combine: Combine the sliced strawberries, blueberries, chopped pineapple, diced mango, and halved grapes in a large mixing dish.
2. Include Cottage Cheese: Fold in the low-fat cottage cheese and mixed fruits gently. Make certain that the distribution is even.
3. Drizzle with honey if desired: To add a touch of sweetness, sprinkle honey over the fruit salad. This is an optional step that can be omitted for a lower sugar content.
4. Optional garnish with mint: Garnish the fruit salad with fresh mint leaves for enhanced freshness and presentation.
5. Serve: Serve the fruit salad immediately in individual serving bowls.

CHAPTER 3: LUNCHTIME FAVORITES

Grilled Chicken Salad:

Ingredients:

- 2 boneless, skinless chicken breasts
- 1 tablespoon olive oil
- 1 teaspoon dried oregano
- 1 teaspoon garlic powder
- Salt and pepper to taste
- 6 cups mixed salad greens (lettuce, spinach, arugula, etc.)
- 1 cup cherry tomatoes, halved
- 1 cucumber, sliced
- 1 red bell pepper, sliced
- 1/2 red onion, thinly sliced
- 1/4 cup feta cheese, crumbled (optional)
- 2 tablespoons balsamic vinaigrette dressing

Preparation Time:20 minutes

Quantity:Serves 2

Instructions:

1. Preheat the grill to medium-high temperature.
2. To make a marinade for the chicken, combine the olive oil, dried oregano, garlic powder, salt, and pepper in a small bowl.
3. Brush the marinade over the chicken breasts, making sure they are uniformly coated.
4. Grill the chicken for 6-8 minutes per side, or until the internal temperature reaches 165°F (74°C) and the center is no longer pink.
5. Prepare the salad while the chicken is grilling by combining the mixed greens, cherry tomatoes, cucumber, red bell pepper, and red onion in a large mixing bowl.
6. Allow the chicken to rest for a few minutes before slicing it into thin pieces.
7. Toss the salad with the grilled chicken strips.
8. If preferred, top the salad with feta cheese.

9. Drizzle the balsamic vinaigrette dressing over the salad and gently toss everything together.

10. Divide the salad between two dishes and serve right away.

Quinoa and Black Bean Bowl:

Ingredients:

- 1 cup quinoa, rinsed
- 2 cups water
- 1 can (15 ounces) black beans, drained and rinsed
- 1 cup cherry tomatoes, halved
- 1 cup cucumber, diced
- 1/2 cup red onion, finely chopped
- 1/4 cup fresh cilantro, chopped
- 1 avocado, sliced
- 1 lime, juiced
- 2 tablespoons olive oil
- 1 teaspoon cumin
- 1/2 teaspoon chili powder
- Salt and pepper to taste

Instructions:

1. Quinoa Cooking: Combine quinoa and water in a medium saucepan.

Bring to a boil, then reduce to a low heat, cover, and cook for 15-20 minutes, or until the quinoa is tender and the water has been absorbed.

With a fork, fluff the quinoa.

2. Prepare the black beans as follows: Warm the black beans in a separate pan over medium heat.

3. Vegetable Mix: Combine the cherry tomatoes, cucumber, red onion, and cilantro in a large mixing basin.

4. Make the dressing: Whisk together lime juice, olive oil, cumin, chili powder, salt, and pepper in a small bowl.

5. Assemble the Bowl: Divide the cooked quinoa across four serving bowls. Black beans, assorted vegetables, and avocado slices go on top.

6. Dressing: Drizzle Pour the lime dressing over the salad.

7. Serve: If preferred, garnish with more cilantro and lime wedges.

Serve and have fun!

Salmon and Vegetable Skewers:

Ingredients:

- 1 pound fresh salmon, cut into 1-inch cubes
- 1 zucchini, sliced into rounds
- 1 red bell pepper, cut into chunks
- 1 yellow bell pepper, cut into chunks
- 1 red onion, cut into wedges
- Cherry tomatoes
- 2 tablespoons olive oil
- 2 cloves garlic, minced
- 1 teaspoon dried oregano
- 1 teaspoon dried thyme
- Salt and pepper to taste
- Lemon wedges for serving

Preparation Time:15 minutes (plus additional time for marinating)

Quantity: Serves 4

Instructions:

1. To make the marinade, combine the olive oil, minced garlic, dried oregano, dried thyme, salt, and pepper in a small bowl.

2. Pour half of the marinade over the salmon cubes in a shallow dish. Toss to coat evenly, then cover and place in the refrigerator for at least 30 minutes to marinate.

3. Prepare the vegetables while the salmon is marinating. Alternately thread the marinated salmon cubes, zucchini slices, bell pepper chunks, red onion wedges, and cherry tomatoes onto skewers.

4. Heat the grill or grill pan to medium-high.

5. Brush the remaining marinade over the skewers.

6. Grill the skewers for 8-10 minutes, flipping halfway through, or until the salmon is cooked through and the veggies are soft.

7. Remove the skewers from the grill and serve with lemon wedges for squeezing over the top.

8. As part of your DASH diet, enjoy your tasty and heart-healthy Salmon and Vegetable Skewers!

Vegetable Stir-Fry with Tofu:

Ingredients:

- 1 block (about 14 ounces) extra-firm tofu, pressed and cubed
- 2 tablespoons low-sodium soy sauce
- 1 tablespoon sesame oil
- 1 tablespoon rice vinegar
- 1 tablespoon fresh ginger, minced
- 2 cloves garlic, minced
- 1 tablespoon olive oil
- 1 medium broccoli crown, cut into florets
- 1 bell pepper (any color), thinly sliced
- 1 medium carrot, julienned
- 1 zucchini, sliced
- 1 cup snap peas, trimmed

- 1 cup mushrooms, sliced
- 2 green onions, sliced
- 1 tablespoon sesame seeds (optional, for garnish)
- Brown rice or quinoa (cooked), for serving

Preparation Time:20 minutes (excluding tofu pressing time)

Quantity:4 servings

Instructions:

1. Tofu should be pressed to remove extra water before cutting into cubes.
2. Tofu cubes should be mixed with soy sauce, sesame oil, rice vinegar, minced ginger, and minced garlic in a bowl. Allow at least 10 minutes for it to marinade.
3. Stir-Fry: In a large skillet or wok, heat the olive oil over medium-high heat.
4. Cook until the marinated tofu cubes are browned on all sides in the skillet. Set aside the tofu from the skillet.

5. Stir-Fry Vegetables: If necessary, add a little more olive oil to the same skillet.

6. Broccoli, bell pepper, carrot, zucchini, snap peas, and mushrooms should all be included. Cook for 5-7 minutes, or until the vegetables are crisp-tender.

7. Combine: Return the cooked tofu and vegetables to the skillet and toss everything together until well incorporated.

8. Finish: Sprinkle the stir-fry with chopped green onions and sesame seeds.

9. Serve the stir-fry vegetables over cooked brown rice or quinoa.

Mediterranean Chickpea Salad:

Ingredients:

- 2 cups cooked chickpeas (canned, drained, and rinsed)
- 1 cup cherry tomatoes, halved
- 1 cucumber, diced
- 1/2 red onion, finely chopped

- 1/2 cup Kalamata olives, sliced
- 1/2 cup crumbled feta cheese (optional)
- 1/4 cup extra virgin olive oil
- 2 tablespoons red wine vinegar
- 1 teaspoon dried oregano
- Salt and pepper to taste
- Fresh parsley, chopped (for garnish)

Preparation Time: 15 minutes

Quantity: Serves 4

Instructions:

1. In a large mixing bowl, add the cooked chickpeas, cherry tomatoes, cucumber, red onion, Kalamata olives, and feta cheese (if using).
2. In a small mixing bowl, combine the extra virgin olive oil, red wine vinegar, dried oregano, salt, and pepper.
3. Pour the dressing over the chickpea mixture and gently toss to coat all of the ingredients equally.
4. Allow the salad to marinade in the refrigerator for at least 10 minutes to allow the flavors to mingle.

5. Garnish with fresh chopped parsley just before serving.

6. Serve chilled and enjoy your wonderful and heart-healthy Mediterranean Chickpea Salad!

Turkey and Avocado Wrap:

Ingredients:

- 1 pound turkey breast, thinly sliced
- 4 whole-grain wraps or tortillas
- 2 avocados, sliced
- 1 cup cherry tomatoes, halved
- 1 cup fresh spinach leaves
- 1/2 cup red onion, thinly sliced
- 1/4 cup feta cheese, crumbled
- 1/4 cup plain Greek yogurt
- 2 tablespoons lime juice
- 1 tablespoon olive oil
- 1 teaspoon Dijon mustard
- Salt and pepper to taste

Preparation Time:20 minutes

Quantity:4 servings

Instructions:

1. To make the dressing, whisk together the Greek yogurt, lime juice, olive oil, Dijon mustard, salt, and pepper in a small bowl. Place aside.
2. Place the tortillas or wraps on a clean surface.
3. Place the sliced turkey in the center of each wrap and distribute evenly.
4. Layer avocado slices, cherry tomatoes, spinach leaves, red onion, and crumbled feta cheese on top of the turkey.
5. Drizzle the dressing over each wrap's ingredients.
6. Fold the wrappers in half and roll them up securely, fastening with toothpicks if necessary.
7. Enjoy your tasty and healthful Turkey and Avocado Wraps right away!

Sweet Potato and Lentil Stew:

Ingredients:

- 1 cup dried brown lentils, rinsed and drained
- 2 large sweet potatoes, peeled and diced

- 1 onion, finely chopped
- 2 cloves garlic, minced
- 1 can (14 oz) diced tomatoes, undrained
- 4 cups low-sodium vegetable broth
- 1 teaspoon ground cumin
- 1 teaspoon ground coriander
- 1/2 teaspoon smoked paprika
- Salt and pepper to taste
- 2 tablespoons olive oil
- Fresh parsley for garnish (optional)

Preparation Time:15 minutes prep time

45 minutes cooking time

Quantity: Serves 4

Instructions:

1. Warm the olive oil in a big pot over medium heat. Sauté the onions and garlic until softened.

2. Cook for another 5 minutes, stirring regularly, after adding the diced sweet potatoes to the saucepan.

3. Stir in the ground cumin, coriander, and smoked paprika, covering the vegetables evenly.
4. To the pot, add washed lentils, diced tomatoes (with juice), and vegetable broth. Season to taste with salt and pepper.
5. Bring the stew to a boil, then reduce to a low heat, cover, and cook for 35-40 minutes, or until the lentils and sweet potatoes are cooked.
6. Season with salt and pepper to taste. If the stew becomes too thick, add extra vegetable broth to get the required consistency.
7. Serve the stew hot, garnished if preferred with fresh parsley.

Whole Wheat Pasta with Tomato and Basil:

Ingredients:

- 8 ounces whole wheat pasta
- 2 cups cherry tomatoes, halved
- 1/4 cup fresh basil, chopped

- 2 cloves garlic, minced
- 2 tablespoons olive oil
- 1/4 teaspoon red pepper flakes (optional)
- Salt and pepper to taste
- 1/4 cup grated Parmesan cheese (optional)

Preparation Time:15 minutes

Quantity:4 servings

Instructions:

1. Cook the whole wheat pasta until al dente according to package directions. Set aside after draining.

2. Warm the olive oil in a large skillet over medium heat. Sauté the minced garlic for about 1 minute, or until fragrant.

3. Cook the cherry tomatoes in the skillet for 3-5 minutes, turning regularly, until they soften.

4. If you're using red pepper flakes, add them to the skillet for some more heat. Depending on your preferences, adjust the quantity.

5. Stir in the cooked whole wheat pasta, making sure it's thoroughly coated with the tomato-garlic combination.
6. Season with salt and pepper to taste. Remember that the DASH diet promotes limiting sodium intake, so go easy on the salt.
7. Remove from the fire and stir in the fresh basil.
8. Before serving, sprinkle grated Parmesan cheese over the spaghetti if preferred.
9. Enjoy a tasty and heart-healthy lunch with the Whole Wheat Pasta with Tomato and Basil!

Greek Yogurt Chicken Salad:

Ingredients:

- 2 cups cooked chicken breast, diced
- 1 cup cherry tomatoes, halved
- 1 cucumber, diced
- 1/2 red onion, finely chopped
- 1/2 cup Kalamata olives, pitted and sliced
- 1/2 cup feta cheese, crumbled
- 1/4 cup fresh parsley, chopped

- 1/4 cup extra-virgin olive oil
- 1/4 cup Greek yogurt (low-fat or fat-free)
- 2 tablespoons red wine vinegar
- 1 clove garlic, minced
- 1 teaspoon dried oregano
- Salt and pepper to taste
- Whole grain pita bread (optional, for serving)

Preparation Time:15 minutes

Quantity: Serves 4

Instructions:

1. Combine the chopped chicken, cherry tomatoes, cucumber, red onion, Kalamata olives, feta cheese, and fresh parsley in a large mixing basin.

2. Whisk together the extra-virgin olive oil, Greek yogurt, red wine vinegar, minced garlic, dried oregano, salt, and pepper in a small bowl. Season with salt and pepper to taste.

3. Dress the chicken and vegetable combination with the dressing. Gently toss until everything is uniformly covered in the dressing.

4. Allow the salad to marinade for at least 10 minutes in the refrigerator to allow the flavors to mingle.
5. Toss the salad once more before serving. If desired, serve on a bed of mixed greens or with whole grain pita bread.

Shrimp and Vegetable Brown Rice Bowl:
Ingredients:
- 1 cup brown rice (uncooked)
- 1 pound shrimp, peeled and deveined
- 2 cups broccoli florets
- 1 bell pepper, thinly sliced (any color)
- 1 medium carrot, julienned
- 1 cup snap peas, trimmed
- 3 cloves garlic, minced
- 1 tablespoon olive oil
- 1 teaspoon low-sodium soy sauce
- 1 teaspoon sesame oil
- 1/2 teaspoon ginger, minced
- 1/4 teaspoon black pepper
- 2 green onions, sliced (for garnish)

- 1 tablespoon sesame seeds (for garnish)

Prep Time: 15 minutes

Cooking Time: 30 minutes

Total Time: 45 minutes

Quantity: 4 servings

Instructions:

1. Brown Rice Cooking Instructions: Brown rice should be cooked according to package directions. Place aside.

2. Prepare the shrimp: In a mixing bowl, combine shrimp, garlic, soy sauce, sesame oil, ginger, and black pepper. Allow it to marinade for ten minutes.

3. Vegetable Stir-Fry: Warm the olive oil in a large skillet or wok over medium-high heat. Broccoli, bell pepper, carrot, and snap peas are optional. Cook for 5-7 minutes, or until the vegetables are crisp-tender.

4. How to Cook Shrimp:Place the vegetables on one side of the skillet and the shrimp on the other.

Cook for 2-3 minutes per side, or until the shrimp are pink and opaque.

5. Combine the following ingredients: In the skillet, combine the cooked shrimp and the stir-fried vegetables.

6. Serve: Distribute the cooked brown rice among four serving bowls. Serve the shrimp and veggie combination on top of each bowl.

7. Garnish: Serve with chopped green onions and sesame seeds on top of each bowl.

8. Enjoy: Serve the Shrimp and Vegetable Brown Rice Bowl right away for a tasty, heart-healthy supper!

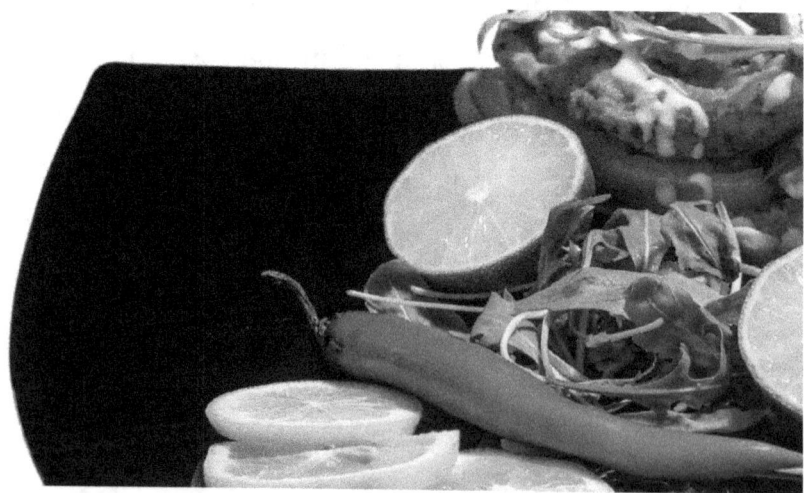

CHAPTER 4: DINNER RECIPES FOR A HEALTHY HEART

Grilled Salmon with Lemon and Herbs:

Ingredients:

- 4 salmon fillets (about 6 ounces each)
- 2 tablespoons olive oil
- 2 tablespoons fresh lemon juice
- 2 teaspoons lemon zest
- 2 cloves garlic, minced
- 1 teaspoon dried oregano
- 1 teaspoon dried thyme
- Salt and pepper to taste
- Lemon slices for garnish
- Fresh parsley, chopped, for garnish

Preparation Time: Marinating time: 30 minutes

Grilling time: 10-12 minutes

Quantity: Serves 4

Instructions:

1. Make the marinade: Whisk together olive oil, lemon juice, lemon zest, minced garlic, dried oregano, dried thyme, salt, and pepper in a small bowl.

2. Marinate the salmon as follows: Fill a small dish or a resealable plastic bag halfway with salmon fillets.Pour the marinade over the salmon, coating each fillet thoroughly. Marinate the salmon in the refrigerator for at least 30 minutes to allow the flavors to infiltrate.

3. Preheat the grill as follows: Preheat the grill to medium-high.

4. Grill the salmon as follows: Remove the salmon from the marinade and drain any excess. Place the salmon fillets on a hot grill. Grill the salmon for 4-6 minutes per side, or until it is cooked to your liking and has excellent grill marks.

5. Serve: Grilled salmon should be garnished with lemon slices and chopped fresh parsley.

Serve immediately and enjoy!

Quinoa and Black Bean Stuffed Peppers:

Ingredients:

- 4 large bell peppers, any color
- 1 cup quinoa, rinsed
- 2 cups black beans, cooked (canned, drained, and rinsed)
- 1 cup corn kernels (fresh or frozen)
- 1 cup diced tomatoes
- 1/2 cup diced red onion
- 1/2 cup chopped fresh cilantro
- 1 teaspoon ground cumin
- 1 teaspoon chili powder
- 1/2 teaspoon garlic powder
- Salt and pepper to taste
- 1 cup low-sodium vegetable broth
- 1 cup shredded low-fat cheddar cheese (optional, for topping)

Preparation Time:20 minutes preparation

30 minutes cooking

Instructions:

Preheat the oven to 350°F.

Preheat the oven to 375 degrees Fahrenheit (190 degrees Celsius).

1. Prepare the peppers as follows: Remove the tops of the bell peppers and remove the seeds and membranes. Fill a baking dish halfway with peppers.

2. Quinoa Cooking Instructions: Combine the quinoa and vegetable broth in a medium saucepan. Bring to a boil, then lower to a low heat, cover, and cook for 15-20 minutes, or until the quinoa is tender and the liquid has been absorbed.

3. Make the filling: Combine the cooked quinoa, black beans, corn, diced tomatoes, red onion, cilantro, cumin, chili powder, garlic powder, salt, and pepper in a large mixing dish. Combine thoroughly.

4. Fill the Peppers: Fill each bell pepper with the quinoa-black bean mixture, carefully pressing down to pack the filling.

5. Bake: Cover the baking dish tightly with foil and bake for 25-30 minutes, or until the peppers are cooked.

6. Optional cheese garnish: Sprinkle shredded cheddar cheese on top of each stuffed pepper during the last 5 minutes of baking if preferred.

7. Serve: Remove from the oven and set aside for a few minutes to cool before serving.

8. Optional garnish: If preferred, garnish with more cilantro or a dollop of Greek yogurt.

Chicken and Vegetable Stir-Fry:

Ingredients:

- 1 pound boneless, skinless chicken breasts, thinly sliced
- 2 cups broccoli florets
- 1 red bell pepper, thinly sliced
- 1 yellow bell pepper, thinly sliced

- 1 cup snap peas, ends trimmed
- 1 carrot, julienned
- 3 cloves garlic, minced
- 1 tablespoon low-sodium soy sauce
- 1 tablespoon olive oil
- 1 teaspoon fresh ginger, grated
- 1 teaspoon sesame oil
- 1/2 teaspoon black pepper
- 2 green onions, sliced (for garnish)
- 2 cups cooked brown rice (optional, for serving)

Prep Time: 15 minutes

Cook Time: 15 minutes

Instructions:

1. In a mixing bowl, combine the sliced chicken, soy sauce, and black pepper. Allow for a 10-minute marinating period.

2. In a large skillet or wok, heat the olive oil over medium-high heat.

3. Stir-fry the marinated chicken in the skillet for 5-7 minutes, or until cooked through. Remove and set aside the cooked chicken from the skillet.

4. If necessary, add a little more olive oil to the same skillet. Stir in the garlic and ginger for about 30 seconds, or until fragrant.

5. To the skillet, add broccoli, bell peppers, snap peas, and julienned carrot. Stir-fry for 5-7 minutes more, or until the vegetables are crisp-tender.

6. Add the sesame oil to the skillet with the cooked chicken. Toss everything together until completely incorporated and thoroughly heated.

7. Garnish with green onions, sliced.

8. If desired, serve over cooked brown rice.

Mediterranean Chickpea Salad:

Ingredients:

- 2 cans (15 oz each) chickpeas, drained and rinsed
- 1 cucumber, diced
- 1 cup cherry tomatoes, halved
- 1/2 red onion, finely diced

- 1/2 cup Kalamata olives, pitted and sliced
- 1/2 cup feta cheese, crumbled
- 1/4 cup fresh parsley, chopped
- 1/4 cup fresh mint, chopped

For the Dressing:

- 1/4 cup extra virgin olive oil
- 2 tablespoons red wine vinegar
- 1 clove garlic, minced
- 1 teaspoon dried oregano
- Salt and black pepper to taste

Preparation Time: 15 minutes

Quantity: 4 servings

Instructions:

1. Combine the chickpeas, cucumber, cherry tomatoes, red onion, Kalamata olives, feta cheese, parsley, and mint in a large mixing basin.

2. To make the dressing, mix together the olive oil, red wine vinegar, minced garlic, dried oregano, salt, and black pepper in a small bowl.

3. Pour the dressing over the chickpea mixture and toss gently until evenly covered.

4. Allow the salad to marinade for at least 30 minutes in the refrigerator to allow the flavors to mingle.

5. Give the salad one more toss before serving, and adjust the seasoning as needed.

6. Enjoy this delicious and heart-healthy Mediterranean Chickpea Salad chilled!

Vegetarian Chili:

Ingredients:

- 2 cans (15 oz each) kidney beans, drained and rinsed
- 1 can (15 oz) black beans, drained and rinsed
- 1 can (15 oz) diced tomatoes, undrained
- 1 cup corn kernels (fresh or frozen)
- 1 large onion, chopped
- 1 bell pepper (any color), chopped
- 2 cloves garlic, minced
- 1 zucchini, diced
- 1 cup carrots, diced

- 1 tablespoon olive oil
- 1 tablespoon chili powder
- 1 teaspoon cumin
- 1/2 teaspoon smoked paprika
- 1/2 teaspoon oregano
- Salt and black pepper to taste
- 4 cups vegetable broth
- 1 cup quinoa, uncooked

Preparation Time: 20 minutes

Quantity: 6 servings

Instructions:

1. Warm the olive oil in a big pot over medium heat. Mix in the onion, bell pepper, and garlic. Sauté the vegetables until they are softened.

2. To the pot, add diced zucchini and carrots. Continue to cook for another 5 minutes.

3. Combine the chili powder, cumin, smoked paprika, oregano, salt, and black pepper in a mixing bowl. Allow the spices to roast and release their flavors for another 2 minutes.

4. Pour in the kidney beans, black beans, diced tomatoes (with juices), corn, vegetable broth, and quinoa. To blend, stir everything together thoroughly.

5. Bring the chili to a boil, then lower to a low heat, cover, and leave to simmer for 15-20 minutes, or until the quinoa is tender and the flavors have merged.

6. Season with salt and pepper to taste. If you want a spicier chili, add a pinch of cayenne pepper.

7. Serve the DASH Diet Vegetarian Chili hot, topped with chopped fresh cilantro or green onions if desired.

Baked Cod with Tomatoes and Olives:

Ingredients:

- 4 cod fillets (about 6 ounces each)
- 2 cups cherry tomatoes, halved
- 1/2 cup Kalamata olives, pitted and sliced
- 2 tablespoons extra-virgin olive oil
- 2 cloves garlic, minced
- 1 teaspoon dried oregano
- 1 teaspoon dried thyme
- 1/2 teaspoon black pepper
- 1/4 teaspoon salt
- 1 lemon, thinly sliced
- Fresh parsley, chopped (for garnish)

Preparation Time: 15 minutes

Cooking Time: 20 minutes

Total Time: 35 minutes

Quantity: Serves 4

Instructions:

1. Preheat the oven to 400 degrees Fahrenheit (200 degrees Celsius).

2. Combine half cherry tomatoes, sliced olives, minced garlic, dried oregano, dried thyme, black pepper, and salt in a mixing dish. Toss with 1 tablespoon of olive oil to coat evenly.

3. In a baking dish, place the fish fillets. Season each fillet with salt and black pepper to taste.

4. Distribute the tomato and olive mixture equally over the fish fillets.

5. Drizzle the remaining tablespoon of olive oil over the top, and top each fillet with lemon slices.

6. Bake for about 20 minutes, or until the fish is opaque and flakes readily with a fork, in a preheated oven.

7. Before serving, garnish with fresh chopped parsley.

Turkey and Vegetable Skewers:

Ingredients:

- 1 pound turkey breast, cut into chunks
- 1 zucchini, sliced
- 1 bell pepper, cut into chunks (any color)

- 1 red onion, cut into chunks
- 1 cup cherry tomatoes
- 2 tablespoons olive oil
- 1 teaspoon dried oregano
- 1 teaspoon garlic powder
- 1 teaspoon onion powder
- Salt and pepper to taste
- Wooden skewers, soaked in water for 30 minutes

Prep Time:15 minutes (plus additional 30 minutes for soaking skewers)

Quantity:4 servings

Instructions:

1. Skewers should be prepared as follows: Soak wooden skewers in water for at least 30 minutes to prevent them from burning while cooking. Warm up your grill or grill pan.

2. Marinate the turkey as follows: Combine the turkey pieces, olive oil, dried oregano, garlic powder, onion powder, salt, and pepper in a mixing bowl. Allow it to sit for at least 10 minutes.

3. Skewers should be assembled as follows: Alternate the marinated turkey chunks with zucchini, bell pepper, red onion, and cherry tomatoes on the skewers.
4. Grill: Place the skewers on the grill or grill pan that has been warmed. Cook, stirring regularly, for about 10-15 minutes, or until the turkey is fully cooked and the vegetables are soft.
5. Serve: Remove the skewers from the grill and set aside for a few minutes to rest. To round up a balanced DASH diet meal, serve the turkey and vegetable skewers with a side of nutritious grains like quinoa or brown rice.

Whole Wheat Pasta with Tomato Sauce and Spinach:

Ingredients:

- 8 ounces whole wheat pasta
- 2 cups fresh spinach, washed and chopped
- 2 cloves garlic, minced

- 1 tablespoon olive oil
- 1 can (14 ounces) crushed tomatoes (preferably no added salt)
- 1 teaspoon dried oregano
- 1 teaspoon dried basil
- 1/2 teaspoon onion powder
- 1/4 teaspoon black pepper
- 1/4 teaspoon red pepper flakes (optional for some heat)
- 1/4 cup grated Parmesan cheese (optional for serving)

Preparation Time:15 minutes

Instructions:

1. Cook Whole Wheat Pasta: Bring a large pot of salted water to a boil. Cook the whole wheat pasta according to the package instructions until al dente. Drain and set aside.
2. Prepare Tomato Sauce: In a large skillet, heat olive oil over medium heat. Add minced garlic and sauté until fragrant (about 1 minute).Pour in the crushed

tomatoes and add dried oregano, dried basil, onion powder, black pepper, and red pepper flakes (if using).Simmer the sauce for 10 minutes, stirring occasionally.

3. Add Spinach: Stir in the chopped spinach and cook until wilted.

4. Combine Pasta and Sauce: Add the cooked whole wheat pasta to the skillet with the tomato and spinach sauce. Toss everything together until the pasta is well coated with the sauce.

5. Serve: Divide the pasta among plates.

6. Optional: Sprinkle with grated Parmesan cheese.

7. Enjoy: Serve immediately and enjoy your delicious and heart-healthy Whole Wheat Pasta with Tomato Sauce and Spinach!

Spinach and Mushroom Quiche:

Ingredients:

- 1 pre-made whole wheat pie crust (look for one with low sodium)

- 1 cup fresh spinach, chopped
- 1 cup mushrooms, sliced
- 1 small onion, finely chopped
- 1 clove garlic, minced
- 1 cup reduced-fat shredded Swiss cheese
- 4 large eggs
- 1 cup skim milk
- 1/2 teaspoon salt (optional, or to taste)
- 1/4 teaspoon black pepper
- 1/4 teaspoon nutmeg (optional)

Preparation Time: 15 minutes (preparing ingredients)

40 minutes (baking time)

5 minutes (resting time)

Quantity: 6 servings

Instructions:

1. Preheat the oven to 375 degrees Fahrenheit (190 degrees Celsius).

2. Sauté the onions in a pan over medium heat until tender and transparent. Cook until the mushrooms are soft, then add the garlic. Cook until the spinach

is wilted, about 5 minutes. Remove from the heat and set aside to cool.

3. Beat the eggs in a mixing bowl. Combine the milk, salt (if using), black pepper, and nutmeg in a mixing bowl. Combine thoroughly.

4. In a pie plate, place the pie dough. Cover the crust with the mushroom, spinach, and onion mixture. Top with the shredded Swiss cheese.

5. Over the vegetables and cheese, pour the egg mixture.

6. Bake for 35-40 minutes, or until the quiche is set and the top is golden brown, in a preheated oven.

7. Remove from the oven and cool for 5 minutes before slicing.

8. Enjoy your tasty and nutritious Spinach and Mushroom Quiche while it's still warm!

Grilled Vegetable and Brown Rice Bowl:

Ingredients:

- 1 cup brown rice
- 2 cups mixed vegetables (e.g., bell peppers, zucchini, cherry tomatoes, red onion)
- 2 tablespoons olive oil
- 1 teaspoon dried oregano
- 1 teaspoon dried thyme
- 1 teaspoon garlic powder
- Salt and pepper to taste
- 1 tablespoon balsamic vinegar
- 1 tablespoon fresh lemon juice
- 2 tablespoons chopped fresh parsley (for garnish)

Preparation Time: 15 minutes (plus time for rice to cook)

Quantity: 4 Servings

Instructions:

1. Brown Rice Cooking Instructions: Brown rice should be cooked according to package directions. Place aside.

2. Vegetable Preparation: Warm up the grill or grill pan. Cut the vegetables into bite-size pieces. Toss the vegetables with olive oil, dried oregano, dried thyme, garlic powder, salt, and pepper in a mixing bowl.

3. Vegetables to grill: Grill the seasoned vegetables, rotating occasionally, until browned and tender. This typically takes 8-10 minutes.

4. Assemble the Bowls: Layer the cooked brown rice and grilled vegetables in serving bowls.

5. Make the dressing: Whisk together the balsamic vinegar and fresh lemon juice in a small bowl. Pour the dressing over the salad dishes.

6. Garnish: To add freshness, top with chopped fresh parsley.

7. Serve: Serve the Grilled Vegetable and Brown Rice Bowls right away for a tasty and heart-healthy lunch!

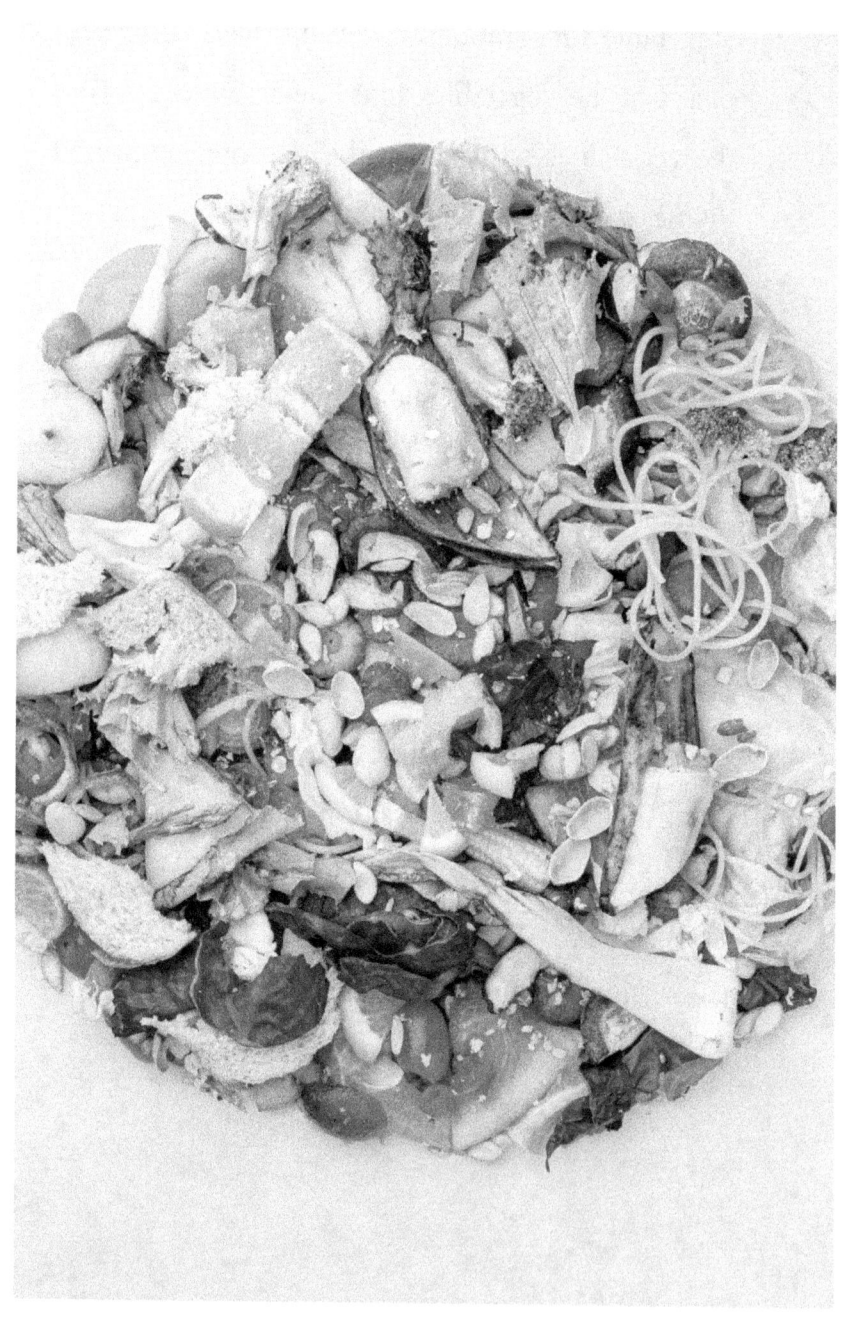

CHAPTER 5: SNACKS AND APPETIZERS

Snacks:

Greek Yogurt Parfait:

Ingredients:

- 1 cup non-fat Greek yogurt
- 1/2 cup fresh berries (blueberries, strawberries, raspberries)
- 1/4 cup granola (low-sugar and whole grain)
- 1 tablespoon honey (optional, for sweetness)
- 1 tablespoon chopped nuts (almonds, walnuts) for added crunch

Preparation Time:10 minutes

Quantity:1 serving

Instructions:

1. Begin with a layer of nonfat Greek yogurt in a glass or bowl.

2. On top of the yogurt, arrange a layer of fresh berries.

3. Sprinkle granola on top of the berries.

4. To add sweetness, sprinkle honey over the granola.

5. Continue layering until you reach the top, finishing with a sprinkle of chopped nuts for texture.

6. Enjoy your tasty and healthful Greek Yogurt Parfait right away!

Hummus with Veggies:

Ingredients:

- 1 can (15 ounces) of chickpeas, drained and rinsed
- 2 cloves garlic, minced
- 1/4 cup tahini
- 1/4 cup extra-virgin olive oil
- 1 teaspoon ground cumin
- 1/2 teaspoon paprika
- Juice of 1 lemon
- Salt and pepper to taste

- Assorted vegetables for dipping (carrot sticks, cucumber slices, bell pepper strips, cherry tomatoes)

Prep Time:10 minutes

Quantity: Makes about 2 cups of hummus

Instructions:

1. Combine chickpeas, minced garlic, tahini, olive oil, cumin, paprika, and lemon juice in a food processor.
2. Scrape down the sides of the bowl as needed to ensure smoothness.
3. Season to taste with salt and pepper. If the hummus is too thick, add a tablespoon of water at a time until it reaches the appropriate consistency.
4. Place the hummus in a serving bowl.
5. Arrange the vegetables for dipping around the hummus.
6. Serve your DASH-friendly Hummus with Veggies and enjoy!

Whole Grain Crackers with Cheese:

Ingredients:

- 1 package of whole grain crackers (look for low-sodium options)
- 1 cup of reduced-fat cheese (such as cheddar, mozzarella, or a blend)
- 1 tablespoon of olive oil
- 1 teaspoon of dried herbs (such as oregano or thyme) for added flavor (optional)
- Fresh vegetables (such as cherry tomatoes or cucumber slices) for garnish (optional)

Preparation Time: 15 minutes

Quantity: Approximately 4 servings

Instructions:

1. Preheat the oven to 350 degrees Fahrenheit (175 degrees Celsius).
2. Arrange the whole grain crackers in a single layer on a baking sheet.
3. Grate the reduced-fat cheese and sprinkle it equally over the crackers.

4. Drizzle a tablespoon of olive oil over the crackers for extra richness.

5. To add flavor, sprinkle dried herbs like oregano or thyme over the cheese (optional).

6. Bake for 5-7 minutes, or until the cheese is melted and bubbling, on a baking sheet in a preheated oven.

7. Remove the crackers from the oven and set aside for a few minutes to cool.

8. If desired, garnish with fresh veggies like as cherry tomatoes or cucumber slices.

9. Serve and savor your heart-healthy Whole Grain Crackers with Cheese!

Fruit Kabobs:

Ingredients:

- 1 cup hulled and halved strawberries
- 1 cup pineapple slices
- 1 cup red or green grapes
- 1 cup watermelon, cubed
- 1 cup cantaloupe, cubed

- 1 cup peeled and sliced kiwi
- Skewers made of wood

To make the dip:

- 1 cup Greek yogurt (nonfat)
- 1 teaspoon honey
- a tsp vanilla extract

Preparation Time: 15 minutes

This recipe yields roughly 6 fruit kabobs.

Instructions:

1. All fruits should be well washed.
2. Remove the hulls from the strawberries and chop them in half.
3. Make bite-sized pineapple chunks.
4. Separate and wash the grapes.
5. Watermelon and cantaloupe should be cut into cubes.
6. Peel and cut the kiwi.
7. Thread the fruits in a bright and pleasing design onto the wooden skewers.

8. To make the dip, combine the Greek yogurt, honey, and vanilla essence in a small bowl.

9. Serve the fruit kabobs beside the yogurt dip.

Nuts Mix:

Ingredients:

- 1 cup almonds
- 1 cup walnuts
- 1/2 cup pistachios (shelled)
- 1/2 cup cashews
- 1/4 cup pumpkin seeds
- 1/4 cup sunflower seeds
- 1 teaspoon olive oil
- 1 teaspoon sea salt (optional, adjust to taste)
- 1/2 teaspoon ground black pepper

Preparation Time: 10 minutes

Quantity: About 3 cups

Instructions:

1. Preheat the oven to 325 degrees Fahrenheit (163 degrees Celsius).

2. Combine almonds, walnuts, pistachios, cashews, pumpkin seeds, and sunflower seeds in a large mixing dish.
3. Drizzle olive oil over the nuts and seeds and toss to coat evenly.
4. Toss with sea salt (if using) and black pepper to taste.
5. Spread the mixture evenly on a parchment-lined baking sheet.
6. Roast for 8-10 minutes, or until the nuts are gently brown and fragrant, in a preheated oven. Keep an eye on them to prevent them from burning.
7. Remove from the oven and cool completely before transferring to an airtight container to store.

Cottage Cheese with Pineapple:
Ingredients:
- 1 cup low-fat cottage cheese
- 1 cup fresh pineapple chunks (or canned pineapple in natural juice, drained)

Optional Add-ins:

- 1 tablespoon chopped mint leaves
- 1 tablespoon chopped walnuts or almonds

Preparation Time:10 minutes

Quantity:2 servings

Instructions:

1. Combine the low-fat cottage cheese and fresh pineapple pieces in a mixing basin.

2. Toss the ingredients together gently until well combined.

3. For a refreshing flavor, add chopped mint leaves if preferred.

4. Sprinkle chopped walnuts or almonds on top for extra crunch and nutrients.

5. Enjoy this healthy and delicious DASH-friendly snack or light meal right away!

Edamame:

Ingredients:

- 2 cups frozen edamame, shelled

- 1 cup cherry tomatoes, halved
- 1/2 cucumber, diced
- 1/4 cup red onion, finely chopped
- 1/4 cup fresh cilantro, chopped
- 2 tablespoons extra virgin olive oil
- 1 tablespoon balsamic vinegar
- 1 clove garlic, minced
- 1/2 teaspoon salt (optional)
- 1/4 teaspoon black pepper
- 1/4 teaspoon red pepper flakes (optional)

Preparation Time: 15 minutes

Quantity: 4 servings

Instructions:

1. Cook the edamame as directed on the package. Allow them to cool to room temperature after draining.

2. Combine the cooked edamame, cherry tomatoes, cucumber, red onion, and cilantro in a large mixing basin.

3. Whisk together the olive oil, balsamic vinegar, minced garlic, salt (if using), black pepper, and red pepper flakes (if used) in a small bowl.

4. Toss the edamame mixture with the dressing until everything is fully coated.

5. Allow the salad to marinade for at least 30 minutes before serving to allow the flavors to blend.

6. Serve chilled as a delightful and nourishing side dish.

Appetizers:

Stuffed Mushrooms:

Ingredients:

- 16 large mushrooms, cleaned and stems removed
- 1 cup quinoa, cooked
- 1 cup spinach, chopped
- 1/2 cup red bell pepper, diced
- 1/4 cup onion, finely chopped
- 2 cloves garlic, minced
- 1/4 cup feta cheese, crumbled (optional)
- 1 tablespoon olive oil

- 1 teaspoon dried oregano
- Salt and pepper to taste

Prep Time: 20 minutes

Quantity: Makes 16 stuffed mushrooms

Instructions:

1. Preheat the oven to 375 degrees Fahrenheit (190 degrees Celsius).

2. Warm the olive oil in a large skillet over medium heat. Sauté the onion and garlic until tender.

3. To the skillet, add diced red bell pepper and chopped spinach. Cook, stirring occasionally, until the veggies are soft and the spinach has wilted.

4. Combine the cooked quinoa, sautéed vegetables, dried oregano, and feta cheese (if using) in a mixing bowl. Season to taste with salt and pepper. Combine thoroughly.

5. Stuff each mushroom cap with the quinoa and vegetable mixture.

6. Place the stuffed mushrooms on a baking sheet and bake for approximately 15 minutes, or until the mushrooms are soft.

7. Remove from the oven and set aside to cool before serving.

Caprese Skewers:

Ingredients:

- Cherry tomatoes, washed and dried
- Fresh mozzarella balls (bocconcini)
- Fresh basil leaves
- Balsamic glaze
- Olive oil
- Salt and pepper to taste
- Wooden skewers

Prep Time:15 minutes

Quantity:Approximately 20 skewers

Instructions:

1. To begin, prepare the cherry tomatoes. They should be completely washed and dried.

2. Drain and set aside the fresh mozzarella balls.
3. Thread a cherry tomato onto each wooden skewer, followed by a mozzarella ball and a fresh basil leaf. Repeat until the skewer is completely filled.
4. Arrange the skewers assembled on a serving plate.
5. Whisk together the balsamic glaze and olive oil in a small basin. Drizzle the skewers with this mixture.
6. Season the skewers to taste with salt and pepper.
7. Enjoy these delicious and heart-healthy Caprese Skewers right away!

Quinoa Salad Cups:

Ingredients:

- 1 cup quinoa, rinsed
- 2 cups water
- 1 cup cherry tomatoes, halved
- 1 cucumber, diced
- 1 bell pepper, diced (any color)
- 1/4 cup red onion, finely chopped
- 1/4 cup feta cheese, crumbled

- 1/4 cup Kalamata olives, pitted and sliced
- 2 tablespoons fresh parsley, chopped
- 2 tablespoons olive oil
- 1 tablespoon red wine vinegar
- Salt and pepper to taste
- Optional: Grilled chicken or chickpeas for added protein

Preparation Time:15 minutes (plus quinoa cooking time)

Quantity:4 servings

Instructions:

1. Quinoa Cooking Instructions: Combine quinoa and water in a medium saucepan. Bring to a boil, then reduce to a low heat, cover, and cook for 15-20 minutes, or until the quinoa is tender and the water has been absorbed. Allow to cool after fluffing with a fork.

2. Vegetable Preparation: Chop the tomatoes, cucumber, bell pepper, red onion, and parsley while the quinoa is cooking.

3. Salad Assemble: Combine the cooked quinoa, cherry tomatoes, cucumber, bell pepper, red onion, feta cheese, Kalamata olives, and parsley in a large mixing basin.

4. Make the dressing: In a small mixing bowl, combine the olive oil, red wine vinegar, salt, and pepper.

5. Toss and combine: Dress the quinoa and vegetables with the dressing. Toss everything until evenly coated.

6. Serve: Divide the quinoa salad among the individual cups or bowls. If preferred, top with more feta cheese and parsley.

7. Protein Optional: You may top the salad with grilled chicken or chickpeas for extra protein.

8. Enjoy: Enjoy your tasty and healthful Quinoa Salad Cups right away!

Guacamole with Veggie Slices:

Ingredients:

- 3 ripe avocados

- 1 small red onion, finely diced
- 2 cloves garlic, minced
- 1-2 medium tomatoes, diced
- 1 lime, juiced
- 1/4 cup fresh cilantro, chopped
- Salt and pepper to taste
- 1 cup cucumber, sliced
- 1 cup bell peppers (assorted colors), sliced
- 1 cup cherry tomatoes, halved
- Carrot sticks for dipping

Preparation Time:15 minutes

Quantity: Makes about 2 cups of guacamole

Instruction:

1. Cut the avocados in half, remove the pits, and scoop out the meat into a basin.

2. With a fork or potato masher, mash the avocados until smooth but still slightly lumpy.

3. To the mashed avocados, add the diced red onion, minced garlic, diced tomatoes, lime juice, and chopped cilantro. Combine thoroughly.

4. Season the guacamole to taste with salt and pepper. As needed, adjust the lime juice or salt.
5. Cut the cucumber, bell peppers, and cherry tomatoes into sticks or slices to make the veggie slices.
6. Serve the guacamole in a bowl with vegetable pieces and carrot sticks for dipping.

Shrimp Cocktail:

Ingredients:

- 1 pound large shrimp, peeled and deveined
- 1 cup cherry tomatoes, halved
- 1 cucumber, diced
- 1/4 cup red onion, finely chopped
- 2 cloves garlic, minced
- 1/4 cup fresh cilantro, chopped
- Juice of 2 limes
- 1 tablespoon extra-virgin olive oil
- 1/2 teaspoon black pepper
- 1/4 teaspoon salt (optional)
- Dash of hot sauce (optional)

Preparation Time: 15 minutes

Quantity: 4 servings

Instructions:

1. Cook the shrimp as follows: Bring a kettle of water to a rolling boil. Cook for 3-4 minutes, or until the shrimp turn pink and opaque. Drain and set aside to cool.

2. Make the Vegetables: Combine the cherry tomatoes, cucumber, red onion, garlic, and cilantro in a large mixing basin.

3. Prepare the Dressing: Whisk together lime juice, olive oil, black pepper, salt (if using), and spicy sauce (if using) in a small bowl.

4. Combine: Cooked shrimp should be added to the veggie combination. Dress the shrimp and vegetables with the dressing. Toss gently until everything is well covered.

5. Chill before serving: Refrigerate the bowl for at least 30 minutes to let the flavors to mingle. Serve

the chilled shrimp cocktail garnished with more cilantro if desired.

Vegetable Spring Rolls:

Ingredients:

- 8 spring roll wrappers (rice paper)
- 2 cups shredded cabbage
- 1 cup julienned carrots
- 1 cup thinly sliced bell peppers (assorted colors)
- 1 cup bean sprouts
- 1 cup thinly sliced cucumber
- 1/2 cup chopped scallions
- 1/4 cup chopped fresh cilantro
- 1/4 cup chopped fresh mint
- 1 tablespoon sesame oil
- 1 tablespoon low-sodium soy sauce
- 1 tablespoon rice vinegar
- 1 teaspoon grated ginger
- 1 teaspoon minced garlic
- 1 cup cooked and shredded chicken (optional for added protein)

Prep Time: Approximately 20 minutes

Quantity: Makes 8 spring rolls

Instructions:

1. To make the vegetables, add shredded cabbage, julienned carrots, sliced bell peppers, bean sprouts, cucumber, scallions, cilantro, and mint in a large mixing dish.

2. To make the sauce, whisk together sesame oil, soy sauce, rice vinegar, grated ginger, and chopped garlic in a small bowl. Season with salt and pepper to taste.

3. Fill a shallow dish halfway with warm water to prepare the rice paper. Dip each rice paper wrapper in water for about 10-15 seconds, or until soft and malleable.

4. Assemble the Spring Rolls: On a clean surface, place the softened rice paper. Place a portion of the veggie mixture in the center of the wrapper. If desired, top with shredded chicken.

5. Fold in the sides of the wrapper and securely roll it from the bottom to the top, sealing the edge. Rep with each spring roll.

6. Serve each spring roll cut in half diagonally with the prepared dipping sauce.

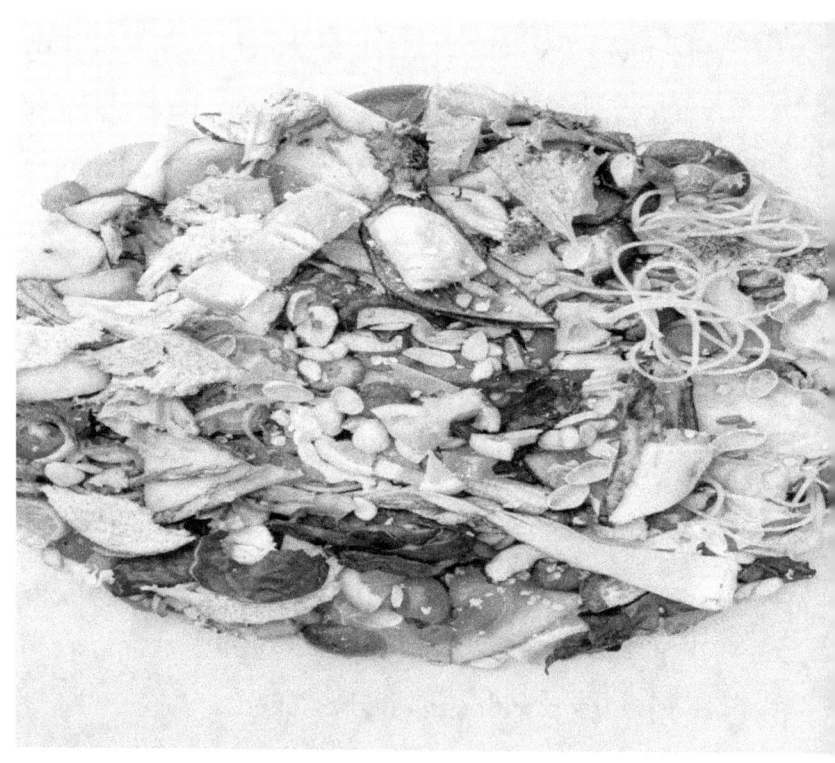

Baked Sweet Potato Fries:

Ingredients:

- 3 medium-sized sweet potatoes, washed and peeled
- 2 tablespoons olive oil
- 1 teaspoon garlic powder
- 1 teaspoon paprika
- 1/2 teaspoon salt (adjust to taste)
- 1/4 teaspoon black pepper
- Optional: 1/2 teaspoon cayenne pepper (for some spice)

Preparation Time: 15 minutes

Quantity: This dish yields 4 servings.

Instructions:

1. Preheat the oven to 425 degrees Fahrenheit (220 degrees Celsius).
2. Cut the sweet potatoes into fries of equal size. To ensure even baking, strive for uniform thickness.
3. Toss the sweet potato fries with olive oil, garlic powder, paprika, salt, black pepper, and cayenne

pepper (if using) in a large mixing bowl. Ensure that the fries are well coated.

4. On a baking sheet, arrange the sweet potato fries in a single layer. To make cleanup easier, use parchment paper.

5. Bake for 25-30 minutes in a preheated oven, rotating the fries midway through to ensure equal cooking. Bake the fries until golden brown and crispy around the edges.

6. Remove from the oven and set aside for a few minutes to cool before serving.

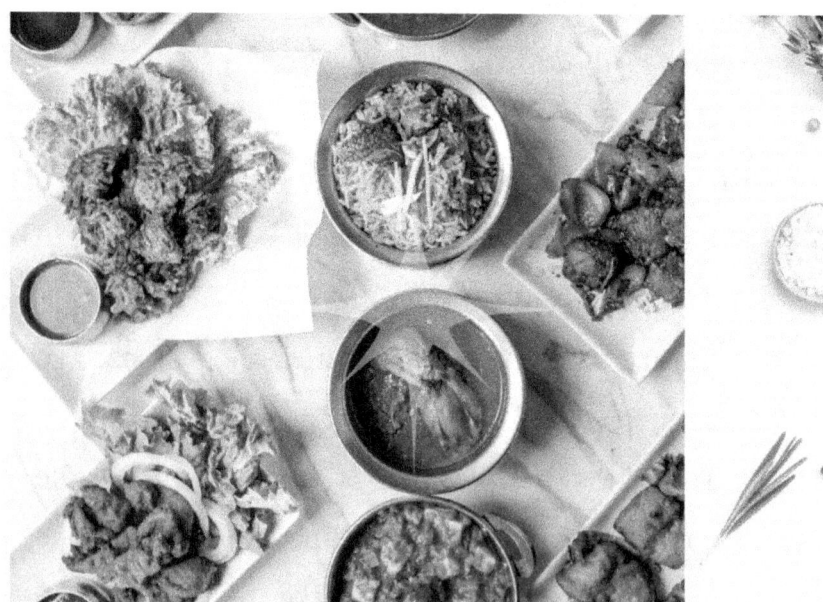

CHAPTER 6: DASH DIET DESSERTS

Mixed Berry Parfait:

Ingredients:

- 1 cup low-fat Greek yogurt
- 1 cup mixed berries (strawberries, blueberries, raspberries)
- 1/4 cup granola (preferably low-sugar)
- 1 tablespoon honey (optional, for sweetness)
- 1/2 teaspoon vanilla extract

Preparation Time:15 minutes

Quantity:2 servings

Instructions:

1. In a mixing dish, combine the Greek yogurt and vanilla essence. If you prefer a sweeter taste, put in some honey with the yogurt.

2. Wash and pat dry the mixed berries well.

3. Begin by putting a dollop of the Greek yogurt mixture on the bottom of serving glasses or bowls.
4. On top of the yogurt, put a layer of mixed berries.
5. Sprinkle granola on top of the berries.
6. Repeat the layers until the glass or bowl is full, concluding with a final layer of berries and a small drizzle of honey if preferred.
7. Rep the previous steps for the second serving.
8. Enjoy your tasty and healthful Mixed Berry Parfait right away!

Chia Seed Pudding:

Ingredients:

- 1/4 cup chia seeds
- 1 cup unsweetened almond milk (or any Dash Diet-approved milk)
- 1/2 teaspoon vanilla extract
- 1 tablespoon honey or maple syrup (optional, adjust to taste)
- Fresh berries (e.g., strawberries, blueberries) for topping

- Chopped nuts (e.g., almonds, walnuts) for topping

Prep Time:5 minutes (plus additional time for chilling)

Quantity:2 servings

Instructions:

1. Combine chia seeds, almond milk, vanilla extract, and honey or maple syrup (if using) in a mixing dish. Stir thoroughly to ensure that the chia seeds are uniformly dispersed.

2. Allow the mixture to sit for a few minutes before stirring again to prevent clumping. Repeat this method a few times more during the next 15 minutes.

3. Refrigerate the bowl for at least 2 hours or overnight to allow the chia seeds to absorb the liquid and form a pudding-like consistency.

4. Give the pudding a good stir before serving. If it's too thick, add a little more almond milk until it's the consistency you want.

5. Top each serving of chia seed pudding with fresh fruit and chopped almonds.

Frozen Banana Bites:

Ingredients:

- 4 ripe bananas
- 1/2 cup Greek yogurt (low-fat)
- 1/4 cup honey
- 1 teaspoon vanilla extract
- 1/2 cup nuts (such as almonds or walnuts), chopped
- 1/4 cup dark chocolate chips (at least 70% cocoa)

Preparation Time: 15 minutes

Quantity: Makes approximately 24 banana bites

Instructions:

1. Peel and cut the bananas into 1-inch thick pieces.
2. Yogurt Concoction: n a mixing dish, combine the Greek yogurt, honey, and vanilla essence.
3. Make the Banana Bites: Dip each banana slice into the yogurt mixture, making sure it is fully coated.
4. Topping with nuts: Roll the coated banana slice in the chopped nuts, ensuring that the nuts adhere to the yogurt.

5. Arrange the following on a tray: Place the coated banana bites on a tray lined with parchment paper, making sure they don't touch.

6. Freeze: Freeze the tray for at least 2 hours, or until the banana bites are totally frozen.

7. Chocolate Melt: In a microwave-safe bowl, melt the dark chocolate chips in 20-second intervals, stirring after each interval, until smooth.

8. Drizzle with chocolate: Melt the chocolate and drizzle it over the frozen banana bites.

9. Last Freeze: Return the tray to the freezer for 30 minutes to allow the chocolate to harden.

10. Serve: Once completely frozen, transfer the banana bites to a freezer-safe container and store in the freezer. Makes a delicious and healthful frozen treat!

Oatmeal and Berry Cookies:

Ingredients:

● 1 cup rolled oats
● 1 cup whole wheat flour

- 1/2 teaspoon baking soda
- 1/2 teaspoon cinnamon
- 1/4 teaspoon salt
- 1/4 cup coconut oil, melted
- 1/4 cup honey or maple syrup
- 1 large egg
- 1 teaspoon vanilla extract
- 1/2 cup mixed berries (blueberries, raspberries, strawberries), fresh or frozen

Preparation Time:15 minutes

Quantity: Makes approximately 2 dozen cookies

Instructions:

1. Preheat the oven to 350 degrees Fahrenheit (175 degrees Celsius) and line a baking sheet with parchment paper.
2. Combine the rolled oats, whole wheat flour, baking soda, cinnamon, and salt in a large mixing basin.

3. Whisk together the melted coconut oil, honey or maple syrup, egg, and vanilla extract in a separate dish until well blended.

4. Mix the wet and dry ingredients together until barely mixed.

5. Fold in the mixed berries gently until they are uniformly distributed throughout the dough.

6. Place rounded portions of dough on a baking sheet lined with parchment paper, about 2 inches apart.

7. Flatten each cookie slightly with the back of a spoon.

8. Bake for 10-12 minutes, or until the edges are golden brown, in a preheated oven.

9. Allow the cookies to cool for 5 minutes on the baking sheet before moving them to a wire rack to cool fully.

10. Enjoy these heart-healthy oatmeal and berry cookies as a nutritious snack or dessert!

Mango Sorbet:

Ingredients:

- 4 cups fresh mango, peeled and diced
- 1/2 cup fresh orange juice
- 1 tablespoon honey (optional, adjust to taste)
- 1 teaspoon lime zest
- 1 tablespoon lime juice

Preparation Time: 15 minutes (plus freezing time)

Quantity: Makes about 4 servings

Instructions:

1. Mango preparation: Remove the pit from fresh mangoes and peel and cube them.

2. Blend: Blend the diced mango, fresh orange juice, honey (if using), lime zest, and lime juice in a blender. Blend until smooth and thoroughly incorporated.

3. Adjust to taste: Taste the mixture and add additional honey if necessary to balance the sweetness.

4. Freeze: Fill a shallow freezer-safe container halfway with the mango mixture. Freeze the sorbet for about 4 hours, or until it is firm.

5. Serve: Allow the sorbet to remain at room temperature for a few minutes before serving to soften slightly. Scoop the sorbet into bowls or cones and serve immediately.

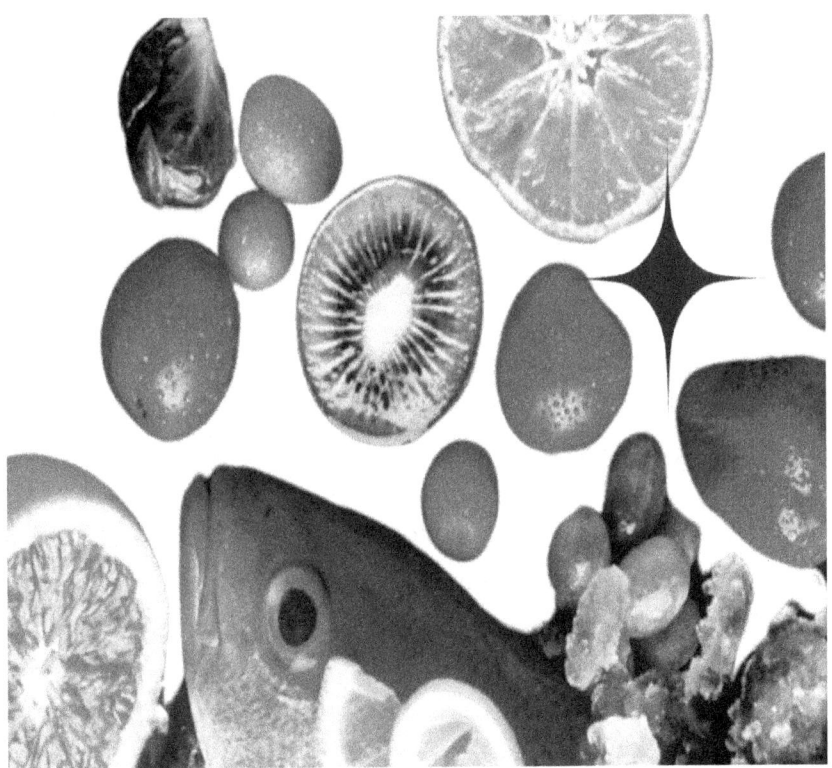

Cinnamon-Spiced Baked Pears:

Ingredients:

- 4 ripe but firm pears, halved and cored
- 1 tablespoon honey (optional, for drizzling)
- 1 teaspoon ground cinnamon
- 1/4 teaspoon ground nutmeg
- 1 tablespoon chopped walnuts or almonds (optional, for garnish)
- Fresh mint leaves, for garnish

Prep Time: 10 minutes

Cook Time: 25 minutes

Total Time: 35 minutes

Quantity: Serves 4

Instructions:

1. Preheat the oven to 375 degrees Fahrenheit (190 degrees Celsius).
2. Place the pear halves cut side up in a baking tray.
3. Combine the cinnamon and nutmeg in a small bowl.

4. Sprinkle the cinnamon-nutmeg mixture over the pear halves, being sure to coat each one equally.

5. If desired, drizzle honey over the pears to add sweetness.

6. Bake for 25 minutes, or until the pears are soft but not mushy, in a preheated oven.

7. Sprinkle chopped nuts over the roasted pears during the last 5 minutes of baking if using.

8. Remove from the oven and let aside to cool somewhat.

9. For a pop of color and taste, garnish with fresh mint leaves.

10. Enjoy this delectable and heart-healthy dessert as part of your DASH diet!

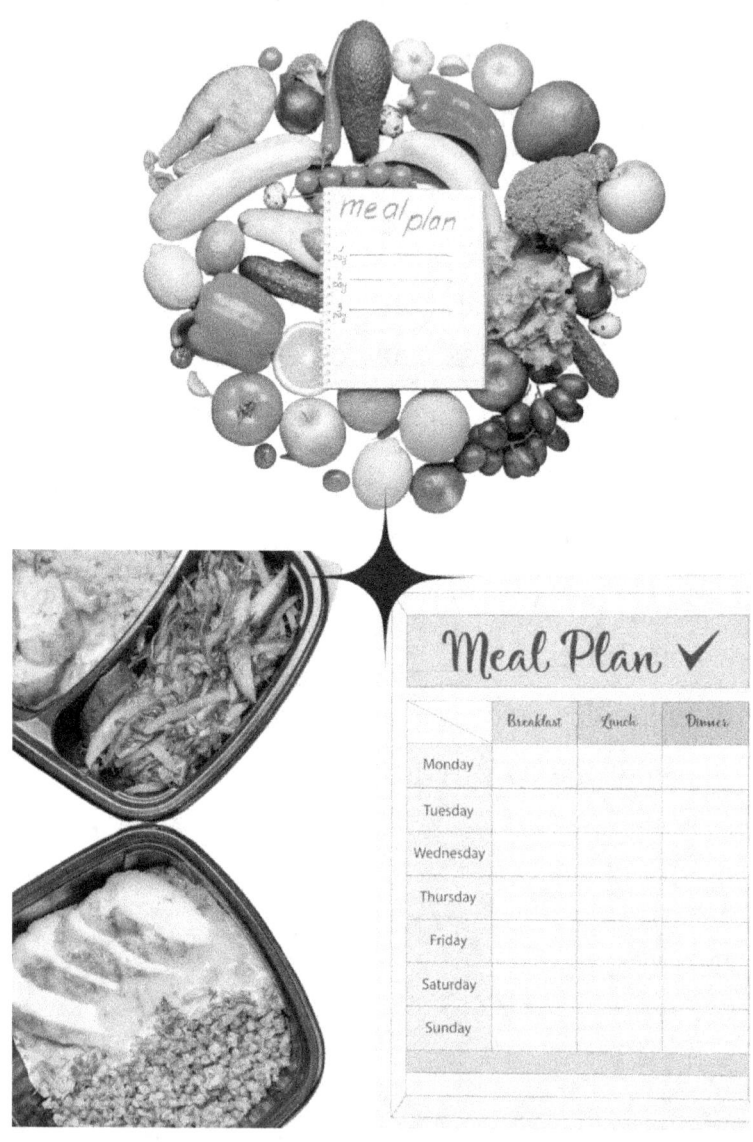

	Breakfast	Lunch	Dinner
Monday			
Tuesday			
Wednesday			
Thursday			
Friday			
Saturday			
Sunday			

CHAPTER 7: BEVERAGES FOR HEART HEALTH

Cucumber Mint Infused Water:

Ingredients:

- 1 medium cucumber, washed and thinly sliced
- 1/4 cup fresh mint leaves, washed
- 1.5 liters (6 cups) of cold water
- Ice cubes (optional)

Preparation Time: 10 minutes

Quantity: Makes approximately 1.5 liters (6 cups) of infused water

Instructions:

1. Wash the cucumber thoroughly before slicing it into thin circles.
2. To unleash the taste of the mint leaves, gently bruise them with the back of a spoon or your fingertips.

3. Combine the sliced cucumber and bruised mint leaves in a big pitcher.
4. Fill the pitcher halfway with cold water, covering the cucumber and mint.
5. To combine the ingredients, carefully stir them together.
6. Allow the infused water to chill for at least 1-2 hours to allow the flavors to mingle.
7. Before serving, add ice cubes if desired.
8. Cucumber Mint Infused Water is delightful when served chilled.

Berry Citrus Smoothie:

Ingredients:
- 1 cup mixed berries (strawberries, blueberries, raspberries)
- 1/2 banana, sliced
- 1/2 cup low-fat yogurt
- 1/2 cup orange juice (freshly squeezed, if possible)
- 1/2 teaspoon honey (optional, for sweetness)
- 1/2 cup ice cubes

Preparation Time:5 minutes

Quantity:2 servings

Instructions:

1. Gather the Ingredients:

Thoroughly wash the berries.

Cut the banana into slices.

2. Combine the following ingredients :Blend together the mixed berries, sliced banana, low-fat yogurt, orange juice, and honey (if used) in a blender. Fill the mixer halfway with ice cubes.

3. Blend until completely smooth: Blend the ingredients on high speed until the mixture is smooth.

4. Thickness can be adjusted: If the smoothie is too thick, add a splash more orange juice and combine until the appropriate consistency is achieved.

5. Serve: Fill the cups with the smoothie. If desired, garnish with a few whole berries on top.

6. Enjoy: Enjoy your cool Berry Citrus Smoothie right away!

Green Tea Lemonade:

Ingredients:

- 4 green tea bags
- 4 cups water
- 2 tablespoons honey (optional, for sweetness)
- 1/2 cup freshly squeezed lemon juice (about 3-4 lemons)
- Ice cubes
- Lemon slices for garnish (optional)
- Mint leaves for garnish (optional)

Prep Time: 10 minutes

Quantity: Makes about 4 servings

Instructions:

1. Boil 4 cups of water and steep the green tea bags in it for 3-5 minutes. Allow it to cool until it reaches room temperature.

2. Remove the tea bags and add honey (if using) once the tea has cooled. Stir until the honey is completely dissolved.

3. Squeeze 1/2 cup fresh lemon juice from the lemons.
4. Combine the green tea and fresh lemon juice in a big pitcher. Stir thoroughly.
5. Fill the pitcher halfway with ice cubes to chill the tea.
6. For a refreshing touch, garnish with lemon slices and mint leaves.
7. Before serving, give the mixture another good stir.

Tomato Basil Gazpacho:
Ingredients:
- 6 medium tomatoes, ripe
- 1 cucumber, peeled and diced
- 1 bell pepper, diced (any color)
- 1 small red onion, finely chopped
- 3 cloves garlic, minced
- 4 cups tomato juice (low-sodium)
- 1/4 cup red wine vinegar
- 1/4 cup extra-virgin olive oil
- 1/2 cup fresh basil leaves, chopped

- Salt and pepper to taste

Preparation Time:15 minutes

Quantity: Serves 4-6

Instructions:

The tomatoes should be peeled and chopped.

Cucumber should be peeled and diced.

Cut the bell pepper into dice.

Chop the red onion finely.

Garlic should be minced.

1. Combine the following ingredients: Combine the chopped tomatoes, diced cucumber, bell pepper, red onion, and minced garlic in a large mixing basin.

2. Blend: Transfer the vegetable mixture to a blender or food processor in batches. Blend each batch with half of the tomato juice until smooth.

3. Season and mix: Return the combined mixture to the large mixing basin. Combine the remaining tomato juice, red wine vinegar, and extra-virgin olive oil in a mixing bowl.Add the basil leaves, chopped. Season to taste with salt and pepper.

4. Chill: Refrigerate the bowl, covered with plastic wrap, for at least 2 hours to allow flavors to mingle.

5. Serve: Pour the cold gazpacho into serving dishes. If desired, garnish with extra basil leaves.

Serve and have fun!

Hibiscus Iced Tea:

Ingredients:

- 4 cups water
- 4 hibiscus tea bags
- 1-2 tablespoons honey or agave syrup (optional, for sweetness)
- 1 lemon, sliced
- Ice cubes (optional)

Preparation Time:10 minutes (plus cooling time)

Quantity: Approximately 4 servings

Instructions:

1. In a kettle or on the stove, bring 4 cups of water to a boil.

2. In a heatproof pitcher, place the hibiscus tea bags.

3. Fill the pitcher halfway with hot water and add the tea bags.

4. Allow the tea to steep for 5-7 minutes, or until it reaches the desired strength.

5. Remove and discard the tea bags.

6. If you like sweetened tea, stir in 1-2 teaspoons honey or agave syrup until it dissolves. To taste, adjust the sweetness.

7. Allow the tea to cool to room temperature before refrigerating it.

8. Add sliced lemon to the iced tea before serving for added flavor.

9. If preferred, serve the hibiscus iced tea over ice cubes.

Pineapple Ginger Smoothie:
Ingredients:
- 1 cup fresh pineapple chunks
- 1/2 inch fresh ginger, peeled and grated
- 1 medium banana

- 1/2 cup Greek yogurt (low-fat or non-fat)
- 1/2 cup skim milk or a dairy-free alternative (e.g., almond milk)
- 1 tablespoon chia seeds
- Ice cubes (optional)
- Honey or maple syrup (optional, for sweetness)

Preparation Time: 10 minutes

Quantity: 2 servings

Instructions:

1. Preparation: Peel and cut the fresh pineapple into slices. Ginger should be peeled and grated. Peel and cut the banana into smaller pieces.
2. Blend the pineapple chunks, grated ginger, banana, Greek yogurt, skim milk (or dairy-free alternative), and chia seeds in a blender. If you want a cooler smoothie, add a handful of ice cubes.
3. Blend the ingredients together until smooth and creamy. If the smoothie is too thick, add more milk or water until the ideal consistency is reached.

4. Taste and Adjust: If necessary, adjust the sweetness of the smoothie. If you like a sweeter flavor, sprinkle with honey or maple syrup.
5. Pour the smoothie into cups and serve right away. If preferred, garnish with a slice of pineapple or a sprinkle of chia seeds.